Breast cancer awareness

Unveiling the Battle Within

George L. Mack

Copyright ©

Table of Contents

9.2 Triumphs and Lessons Learned

10. Conclusion

    10.1 The significance of maintaining breast cancer awareness

    10.2 Encouragement for Early Detection and Support

"Remember, early detection saves lives. Stay informed, spread awareness, and support the fight against breast cancer".

1 | Introduction

Bosom malignant growth also breast cancer is an intricate and pervasive illness that influences a great many individuals around the world. This part expects to give a thorough comprehension of bosom malignant growth, its causes, and the significance of bringing issues to light about it.

1.1 Understanding Breast Cancer

Bosom disease is a kind of malignant growth that starts in the bosom tissue. It happens when unusual cells in the bosom develop and partition wildly, shaping a growth. Bosom malignant growth can influence all kinds of people, despite the fact that it is all the more regularly analyzed in ladies.

To comprehend bosom disease, getting a handle on the construction and capability of the breast is fundamental. The bosom is made out of glandular tissue, conduits that convey milk to the areola, greasy tissue, and veins. Bosom malignant growth can be created in any of these parts.

1.2 Importance of Breast Cancer Awareness

Bosom disease mindfulness assumes an essential part in early location, treatment, and counteraction. By bringing issues to light about bosom malignant growth, people can turn out to be more educated about the infection, its gambling factors, and the significance of normal screenings.

Early identification is vital to further developing bosom malignant growth results. At the point when bosom malignant growth is identified at a beginning phase, treatment choices are more powerful, and the possibilities of endurance increment essentially. Bosom self-assessments, clinical bosom assessments, and mammograms are crucial instruments for early discovery.

Notwithstanding early recognition, bosom malignant growth mindfulness diminishes the disgrace related with the infection. It energizes open discussions about bosom wellbeing, engages people to look for clinical exhortation, and advances encouraging groups of people for those impacted by bosom disease.

Bosom malignant growth mindfulness missions, occasions, and instructive projects assume a crucial part in dispersing exact and forward-thinking data about the sickness. They mean to teach the general population about risk factors, avoidance systems, and accessible assets for help and treatment.

By advancing bosom disease mindfulness, people can add to the general exertion of decreasing the effect of bosom malignant growth on people, families, and networks. It supports proactive wellbeing ways of behaving, enables people to pursue informed choices, and cultivates a feeling of fortitude among those impacted by bosom disease.

Taking everything into account, the presentation segment of this far reaching guide gives an outline of bosom disease and stresses the meaning of bosom malignant growth mindfulness. Understanding bosom malignant growth and bringing issues to light about it can prompt early identification, further developed treatment results, and a strong climate for those impacted by the illness. By effectively partaking in bosom disease mindfulness drives, people can add to the battle against bosom malignant growth and assist with saving lives.

Kindly note that this is only a concise outline of the point. The main subject will jump further into the different parts of grasping bosom malignant growth and the significance of bosom disease mindfulness.

2 | Risk Factors and Prevention

Bosom malignant growth is a perplexing sickness that can influence anybody, paying little mind to progress in years or orientation. While the specific reason for bosom disease is at this point unclear, there are a few gamble factors that have been distinguished. Understanding these gamble factors and going to preventive lengths can altogether lessen the possibilities of bosom disease.

2.1 Genetic and Environmental Factors

One of the most notable gambling factors for bosom malignant growth is a family background of the illness. Ladies who have a first-degree relative (like a mother or sister) with bosom malignant growth have a higher gamble of fostering the actual illness. Furthermore, certain quality changes, like BRCA1 and BRCA2, extraordinarily increment the gamble of bosom disease. Hereditary testing can assist with distinguishing people who are at a higher gamble and consider proper preventive measures.

Natural factors likewise assume a part in bosom malignant growth risk. Openness to specific synthetics, like those tracked down in pesticides, plastics, and beauty care products, may improve the probability of creating bosom malignant growth. It is essential to limit openness to these harmful substances and pick items that are liberated from possibly destructive synthetic compounds.

2.2 Lifestyle Choices and Breast Cancer Risk

A few way of life decisions can impact the gamble of creating bosom disease. Weight, for instance, is related with an expanded gamble of bosom malignant growth, especially in postmenopausal ladies. Keeping a sound load through normal activity and a fair eating routine can assist with lessening this gamble.

Another factor that has been linked to breast cancer is drinking alcohol. Studies have demonstrated the way that even safe liquor utilization can expand the gamble of fostering the infection. Restricting liquor admission or staying away from it through and through can assist with bringing down the gamble.

2.3 Early Detection and Screening

Early recognition assumes an urgent part in the effective therapy of bosom malignant growth. Routine screening tests like Mammograms and others can be used to detect Breast cancer in its earliest stages when it is most treatable. It is suggested that ladies go through customary mammograms beginning at 40 years old, or prior assuming that they have a higher gamble.

Self-exams of the breasts are another important component of early detection. Ladies ought to perform month to month self-tests to get comfortable with the typical look and feel of their bosoms. Any changes, like bumps, dimpling, or areola release, ought to be quickly answered to a medical care proficient.

Notwithstanding normal screenings, it is fundamental to know about the signs and side effects of bosom disease. These may remember a protuberance or thickening for the bosom or underarm region, changes in bosom size or shape, areola changes, or bosom torment. Brief clinical consideration ought to be looked for in the event that any of these side effects are capable.

Avoidance is key with regards to bosom disease. By understanding the gamble factors and pursuing sound way of life decisions, people can altogether diminish their possibilities fostering the sickness. Early discovery and constant screenings are additionally significant for getting bosom disease in its earliest and most treatable stages. Everybody should remain educated, spread mindfulness, and back the battle against bosom malignant growth. Keep in mind, early identification saves lives.

3 | Types and Stages of Breast Cancer

Bosom malignant growth is a mind boggling and different sickness that can appear in different structures and progress through various stages. For accurate diagnosis, treatment planning, and prognosis, it is essential to understand the various types and stages of breast cancer. In this part, we'll talk about the many forms of breast cancer and their phases of development.

3.1 Non-invasive Breast cancer

Non-invasive Breast Cancer, otherwise called carcinoma in situ, alludes to unusual cells that are restricted to the milk channels or lobules of the bosom and have not spread to encompassing tissues. DCIS (Ductal carcinoma in situ) and LCIS (lobular carcinoma in situ) are the two most common types of benign breast malignancy. DCIS is the most well-known type and is described by strange cells inside the milk channels. LCIS, then again, includes unusual cells inside the lobules.The beginning phase of harmless bosom malignant growth is profoundly treatable and has a high endurance rate.

3.2 Invasive Breast cancer

Invasive Breast Cancer, otherwise called penetrating bosom malignant growth, happens when strange cells get through the pipes or lobules and attack encompassing bosom tissue. Based on the type of cells involved, this type of breast cancer is further divided into several subtypes. The most well-known sorts of invasive breast cancer are invasive ductal carcinoma (IDC), invasive lobular carcinoma (ILC), and inflammatory breast cancer (IBC).

- <u>Invasive Ductal Carcinoma (IDC)</u>: IDC is the most well-known sort of invasive breast cancer, representing around 70-80% of all cases.

- <u>Invasive Lobular Carcinoma (ILC)</u>: ILC, which develops in the breast lobules, accounts for around 10-15% of invasive breast malignancies. It will in general be less characterized and harder to recognize on imaging tests contrasted with IDC.

- <u>inflammatory breast cancer (IBC)</u>: About 1% to 5% of cases of breast cancer are characterized by IBC, a rare and aggressive form.Due to the breast's redness, swelling, and tenderness, it mimics an infection. IBC requires quick clinical consideration and serious treatment.

3.3 Staging and Prognosis

Bosom malignant growth organizing is a framework used to portray the degree and spread of the illness. The most ordinarily utilized organizing framework is the TNM framework, which represents cancer, lymph nodes, and metastasis.

- <u>Tumor, or T</u>: The T classification depicts the size and degree of the essential cancer. It goes from T0 (no proof of a cancer) to T4 (huge growth with broad intrusion of encompassing tissues).

- <u>Lymph Nodes (N)</u>: The N class shows whether malignant growth has spread to local lymph nodes. It goes from N0 (no disease in the lymph node) to N3 (broad malignant growth contribution in different lymph nodes).

- <u>Metastasis (M)</u>: The presence or absence of distant metastasis, which indicates cancer spreading to other parts of the body, is referred to as the M category. It is classified as M0 (no far off metastasis) or M1 (far off metastasis present).

In light of the TNM arranging, bosom malignant growth is additionally grouped into four fundamental stages:

- <u>Stage 0</u>: This stage alludes to harmless bosom malignant growth, like DCIS or LCIS, where strange cells are bound to the milk pipes or lobules.

- <u>Stage I</u>: The tumor is small, confined to the breast, and does not involve any lymph nodes at this stage.

- <u>Stage II</u>: This stage is separated into IIA and IIB. In stage IIA, the cancer is still little yet may include close by lymph hubs. In stage IIB, the growth might be bigger or include various lymph hubs.

- <u>Stage III</u>: According to research, stage III is further divided into IIIA, IIIB, and IIIC.

In these stages, the cancer is bigger, may include different lymph hubs, and may have spread to the chest wall or skin.

- <u>Stage IV</u>: This stage shows metastatic bosom disease, where malignant growth has spread to far off organs or tissues, like the lungs, liver, bones, or mind.

The phase of bosom malignant growth assumes a huge part in deciding treatment choices and foreseeing guesses. While advanced-stage breast cancer (stages III and IV) may require more aggressive treatments and have a lower overall survival rate, early-stage breast cancer (stages 0 to II) generally has a higher chance of successful treatment and long-term survival.

All in all, bosom disease envelops different sorts and stages, each with its own attributes and suggestions for treatment and anticipation. Early recognition through ordinary screenings and familiarity with the signs and side effects are fundamental in further developing results. Individuals can support efforts to raise awareness and promote early detection of breast cancer by having a solid understanding of its stages and types.

4 | Symptoms and Diagnosis

4.1 Common Symptoms of Breast Cancer

Breast cancer can present with various symptoms, although it's important to note that not all individuals will experience noticeable symptoms. Common breast cancer symptoms include:

- A knot or thickening in the bosom or underarm region

- Changes in bosom size or shape
- Areola changes, like reversal, release, or scaling.
- Skin changes on the breast, such as redness, dimpling, or puckering
- Breast pain or tenderness

It's important to remember that these symptoms can also be caused by non-cancerous conditions, such as cysts or infections. However, if any of these symptoms persist or are concerning, it is essential to consult a healthcare professional for further evaluation.

4.2 Diagnostic Tests and Procedures

If breast cancer is suspected based on symptoms or screening tests, further diagnostic tests and procedures may be recommended. These may consist of:

- <u>Mammogram</u>: A mammogram is an X-ray of the breast that is used to look for anomalies that might be signs of breast cancer, such as tumors or calcifications.

- <u>Ultrasound</u>: Sound waves are used by an ultrasound to create images of the breast tissue. It may assist in determining whether a breast lump is solid or cystic, or filled with fluid.

- <u>Magnetic Resonance Imaging (MRI)</u>: A MRI utilizes a magnetic field and radio waves to make itemized pictures of the bosom. It can give extra data about the degree of the illness.

- Biopsy: A biopsy involves the removal of a sample of breast tissue for further examination under a microscope. This is the most conclusive method for diagnosing bosom disease.

- <u>Blood tests</u>: Blood tests might be performed to assess specific markers, for example, chemical receptor status or hereditary transformations, that can assist with directing treatment choices.

The specific tests and procedures recommended will depend on various factors, including the individual's age, medical history, and the characteristics of the breast abnormality.

It is important to remember that the presence of symptoms or abnormal findings does not necessarily mean a diagnosis of breast cancer. Only a healthcare professional can make an accurate diagnosis based on a combination of clinical evaluation, imaging studies, and biopsy results.

5 | Treatment Alternatives for Breast Cancer

The treatment of breast cancer is complex and requires a variety of approaches. In this section, we will investigate different therapy options accessible for people tested with bosom malignant growth. We will examine the options that give patients the ability to make informed decisions about their healing and recovery journey, including surgical interventions and targeted therapies.

5.1 Medical procedure: Lumpectomy and Mastectomy

Medical procedure assumes an essential part in the administration of bosom disease. Two essential careful choices are normally utilized: lumpectomy and mastectomy. Lumpectomy includes the evacuation of the growth and a little piece of surrounding healthy tissue, safeguarding the bosom however much as could reasonably be expected. Mastectomy, then again, includes the total expulsion of the bosom tissue. Each approach has its advantages and contemplations, and the choice ought to be made in discussion with medical care experts.

5.2 Radiation Treatment

Radiation treatment uses high-energy X-beams or other particles to annihilate malignant growth cells/cancer cells and lessen the gamble of repetition. Post-surgery, it is frequently utilized to target any remaining breast cancer cells or lymph nodes. Radiation treatment is a localized treatment that aims to limit damage to sound tissues while successfully focusing on malignant growth cells.

5.3 Chemotherapy

Chemotherapy involves the administration of potent drugs to the body to eradicate cancer cells. It is administered either intravenously or orally, permitting the drug to flow in the circulatory system and arrive at cancer cells in different parts of the body. Chemotherapy can be used either before or after surgery for people with aggressive or advanced breast cancer.

5.4 Targeted Therapy

A treatment strategy that focuses on specific molecular changes in cancer cells is called targeted therapy. By focusing on these particular changes, designated treatments can upset cancer cell development and survival while limiting harm to healthy cells. This approach has shown promising outcomes in treating specific kinds of bosom disease, like HER2-positive bosom malignant growth.

5.5 Hormone Therapy

Patients with hormone receptor-positive breast cancer typically benefit most from hormone therapy. It works by obstructing or diminishing the impacts of hormones, for example, estrogen and progesterone, which can invigorate the development of hormone receptor-positive bosom disease cells. Hormone Therapy can be administered orally or through injections, and its term might differ depending upon individual conditions.

By investigating these treatment choices, people can acquire a more profound comprehension of the choices accessible to them. It is vital to take note that therapy choices ought to be made as a team with medical care experts, considering different factors like the phase of malignant growth, individual preferences, and potential side effects.

Engaging patients with information about treatment choices empowers them to effectively partake in their recuperating and recuperation process. It encourages a feeling of control and assists people with pursuing informed choices that line up with their qualities and objectives. With headways in clinical exploration and customized medication, the scene of bosom malignant growth treatment keeps on advancing, offering trust and further developed results for patients.

All in all, therapy choices for bosom malignant growth give patients a scope of choices to consider on their recuperating and recuperation venture. From careful intercessions to designated treatments, each approach has its advantages and contemplations. Individuals can actively participate in their treatment decisions by comprehending these options, enabling them to navigate their breast cancer journey with confidence and resilience.

6 | Coping with Breast Cancer

Breast cancer is a struggle that involves not only physical but also psychological and emotional aspects. Coping with the diagnosis and the subsequent treatment can be overwhelming, but there are various strategies and support systems available to help individuals navigate through this challenging journey.

6.1 Emotional and Psychological Effects

The emotional and psychological effects of breast cancer can vary from person to person. It is normal to experience a range of emotions such as fear, anxiety, sadness, anger, and even grief. Coping with these emotions is crucial for overall well-being.

The use of expert assistance is one efficient means of controlling these feelings. Psychologists and counselors with experience in oncology can provide a safe space for individuals to express their feelings and help them develop coping strategies. Additionally, joining support groups or online communities specifically for breast cancer patients can be immensely beneficial. These platforms provide an opportunity to connect with others who are going through or have gone through similar experiences, fostering a sense of understanding, empathy, and shared strength.

6.2 Support Systems and Resources

Building a strong support system is essential when coping with breast cancer. Friends, family, and loved ones can offer emotional support, accompany individuals to medical appointments, and provide practical assistance with daily tasks. It is important to communicate openly with them about needs, concerns, and boundaries to ensure effective support.

In addition to personal networks, there are numerous resources available to breast cancer patients. Cancer support organizations, such as the American Cancer Society and Susan G. Komen, offer a wealth of information, support services, and helplines. These organizations often provide educational materials, financial assistance, transportation services, and access to support groups.

6.3 Self-Care and Wellbeing

Taking care of oneself during the breast cancer journey is vital. Self-care practices can help manage stress, improve overall well-being, and enhance the ability to cope with the challenges of treatment. Some self-care strategies include:

a) <u>Physical well-being</u>: Engaging in regular exercise, maintaining a healthy diet, and getting enough rest can contribute to physical strength and overall well-being. It is important to consult healthcare providers for guidance on exercise and nutrition during treatment.

b) <u>Mindfulness and relaxation techniques</u>: Practices such as meditation, deep breathing exercises, and yoga can help reduce anxiety and promote a sense of calmness. These techniques can be learned through classes, online resources, or apps.

c) <u>Expressive therapies</u>: Engaging in creative activities such as art, music, or writing can provide an outlet for emotions and serve as a form of self-expression. These activities can be done individually or as part of therapy programs.

d) <u>Maintaining social connections</u>: Staying connected with loved ones and participating in social activities can help combat feelings of isolation and provide a sense of normalcy. However, it is important to respect personal boundaries and prioritize self-care when needed.

e) <u>Seeking joy and laughter</u>: Engaging in activities that bring joy, laughter, and a sense of normalcy can be incredibly uplifting. This can include watching comedies, spending time with loved ones, or pursuing hobbies and interests.

In conclusion, coping with breast cancer involves addressing the emotional and psychological effects, building a support system, and prioritizing self-care. Seeking professional help, joining support groups, and utilizing available resources can provide individuals with the necessary tools to navigate through this challenging journey. By focusing on emotional well-being, accessing support systems, and practicing self-care, individuals can enhance their overall quality of life and resilience during and after breast cancer treatment.

7 | Survivorship and Beyond

Survivorship is a significant milestone for individuals who have completed breast cancer treatment. However, life after treatment brings its own set of challenges and adjustments. This section explores various aspects of survivorship, including post-treatment life, long-term side effects, follow-up care, and the importance of advocacy and breast cancer awareness campaigns.

7.1 Life After Breast Cancer Treatment

Completing breast cancer treatment marks the beginning of a new chapter in a person's life. It is important to acknowledge that the transition from active treatment to survivorship can be emotionally and psychologically complex. Many individuals experience a mix of emotions, including relief, gratitude, and uncertainty about the future.

During this phase, it is crucial to establish a new sense of normalcy and focus on rebuilding physical and emotional well-being. Regular follow-up appointments with healthcare providers are essential to monitor any potential recurrence or new health concerns. These appointments may include physical examinations, imaging tests, and blood work. It is important to communicate openly with healthcare providers about any symptoms or concerns that arise.

Reintegrating into daily life and resuming activities that were put on hold during treatment can be both exciting and challenging. It is essential to pace oneself and listen to the body's needs. Gradually returning to work, hobbies, and social activities can help restore a sense of purpose and normalcy. However, it's crucial to emphasize self-care and set achievable objectives.

Family support continues to be essential during the surviving period. Friends and family may offer moral support, assistance with daily duties, and encouragement. Participating in internet-based forums or support networks for breast cancer survivors can also be beneficial.

 These platforms offer a space to share experiences, gain insights, and connect with others who have gone through similar journeys.

7.2 Long-Term Side Effects and Follow-Up Care

While completing breast cancer treatment is a significant achievement, it is important to be aware of potential

long-term side effects that may arise.
Depending on the type of therapy taken
and personal characteristics, these side
effects might change. Fatigue,
lymphedema, menopausal symptoms,
cognitive problems, and emotional
anguish are examples of frequent
long-term adverse effects.

The usual adverse effect of fatigue is that
it might linger even after therapy. Putting
rest first, exercising frequently, and
controlling stress can all assist with
tiredness management. Lymph node
excision or radiation therapy may result in
lymphedema, a disorder marked by
swelling in the arm or chest. Lymphedema
may be controlled by taking precautions

like avoiding heavy lifting and wearing compression clothing.

Many breast cancer therapies might hasten or cause menopausal symptoms. Vaginal dryness, mood swings, and heat flashes are a few examples of these symptoms.

 Discussing these symptoms with healthcare providers can help explore management strategies, such as hormone replacement therapy or non-hormonal interventions.

Cognitive changes, often referred to as "chemo brain," can affect memory, concentration, and overall cognitive function. Engaging in mental exercises, maintaining a healthy lifestyle, and seeking support from healthcare providers can help manage these changes.

Emotional distress, including anxiety and depression, can persist even after treatment. Seeking support from mental health professionals, participating in counseling or therapy, and engaging in stress-reducing activities can aid in emotional well-being.

Follow-up care plays a crucial role in monitoring for any potential recurrence or new health concerns. Regular check-ups, mammograms, and other imaging tests are essential components of follow-up care. It is important to communicate openly with healthcare providers about any symptoms or concerns that arise between appointments. Maintaining a healthy lifestyle, including regular exercise, a balanced diet, and avoiding tobacco and excessive alcohol use, can also contribute to overall well-being and reduce the risk of recurrence.

7.3 Advocacy and Breast Cancer Awareness Campaigns

Breast cancer survivors have a unique perspective and voice in raising awareness about the disease and advocating for change. By sharing personal experiences and insights, survivors can help educate others, promote early detection, and support those currently facing breast cancer.

Advocacy can take various forms, from participating in awareness campaigns and fundraising events to sharing personal stories through social media or traditional media outlets. Engaging with local and national breast cancer organizations can provide opportunities to contribute to research, support programs, and policy initiatives.

Survivors can also support and empower others by providing information and resources, participating in support groups, and volunteering their time and expertise. By offering a listening ear, sharing experiences, and providing emotional support, survivors can make a significant impact on the lives of others facing breast cancer.

In conclusion, survivorship is a significant milestone, but it comes with its own set of challenges and adjustments. Life after breast cancer treatment involves establishing a new sense of normalcy, managing potential long-term side effects, and prioritizing follow-up care. By sharing personal experiences and engaging in advocacy efforts, survivors can contribute to raising awareness, supporting others, and promoting positive change in the fight against breast cancer.

8 | Promoting Breast Cancer Awareness

Breast cancer is a global health concern that affects millions of women and men every year. Promoting breast cancer awareness is crucial in raising public understanding, encouraging early detection, and supporting those affected by the disease. This section will delve into various strategies and initiatives aimed at promoting breast cancer awareness, including community outreach programs, fundraising and support initiatives, and spreading awareness through education.

8.1 Community Outreach Programs

Community outreach programs play a vital role in promoting breast cancer awareness at the grassroots level. These programs involve engaging with local communities, organizing events, and providing education and resources to increase knowledge about breast cancer. One effective approach is hosting awareness campaigns in collaboration with healthcare professionals, local organizations, and volunteers. These campaigns can include informative talks, interactive workshops, and free screening services.

Additionally, community outreach programs can focus on reaching underserved populations, such as low-income communities, rural areas, and minority groups. By tailoring outreach efforts to address specific cultural, linguistic, and socioeconomic barriers, these programs can ensure that all individuals have access to vital information about breast cancer prevention, early detection, and treatment options.

Another important aspect of community outreach programs is the establishment of support networks. For those impacted by breast cancer, these networks can provide emotional support, significant help, and an aura of community. Support groups, helplines, and online forums are some examples of resources that can be made available through community outreach programs. By connecting individuals with similar experiences, these networks can help reduce feelings of isolation and provide a platform for sharing stories, advice, and encouragement.

8.2 Fundraising and Support Initiatives

Fundraising initiatives are essential for supporting research, treatment, and support services for breast cancer patients. These initiatives can take various forms, such as charity runs, walks, and other community events.

Engaging the community in these activities not only raises funds but also fosters a sense of unity and solidarity in the fight against breast cancer.

In addition to community events, fundraising campaigns can be organized through online platforms, allowing individuals from different locations to contribute to the cause. Crowdfunding websites, social media campaigns, and virtual events have become increasingly popular in recent years, enabling individuals to make donations or participate in fundraising activities from the comfort of their own homes.

Furthermore, support initiatives are crucial for individuals affected by breast cancer.

Support groups provide a safe space for patients, survivors, and their loved ones to share experiences, seek emotional support, and exchange information. These groups can be organized through hospitals, community centers, or online platforms, allowing individuals to connect with others who understand their journey.

Support initiatives can also include counseling services, educational resources, and practical assistance. By providing comprehensive support, individuals affected by breast cancer can better cope with the emotional, physical, and financial challenges that may arise during their journey.

8.3 Spreading Awareness through Education

Education is a powerful tool in promoting breast cancer awareness. By providing accurate and up-to-date information, educational initiatives can empower individuals to make informed decisions about their health. Schools, workplaces, and community centers can host workshops and seminars to educate people about breast cancer risk factors, early signs, and the importance of regular screenings.

In addition to in-person events, utilizing digital platforms is an effective way to reach a wider audience. Social media campaigns, websites, and online resources can provide accessible information about breast cancer prevention, self-examination techniques, and available support services. These platforms also facilitate the sharing of personal stories, inspiring others and fostering a sense of community.

Collaboration with healthcare professionals, researchers, and advocacy organizations is key to ensuring the accuracy and relevance of educational materials. By working together, these stakeholders can develop evidence-based resources that address the specific needs and concerns of different populations.

Conclusion

Promoting breast cancer awareness is a collective effort that requires the involvement of individuals, communities, and organizations. Community outreach programs, fundraising initiatives, and spreading awareness through education are key components in this endeavor. By engaging with local communities, providing support services, and disseminating accurate information, we can empower individuals to take proactive steps in preventing breast cancer and supporting those affected by the disease.

Remember, that promoting breast cancer awareness is not only about raising public knowledge but also about creating a supportive and compassionate environment for patients and survivors. Together, let us continue to spread awareness, support research, and advocate for early detection, as early detection saves lives.

9 | Inspiring Stories of Hope and Resilience

Breast cancer is a challenging journey that affects millions of individuals worldwide. Amidst the difficulties and uncertainties, there are stories of hope and resilience that inspire and uplift those facing this disease. In this section, we will explore personal accounts of breast cancer survivors, their triumphs, and the lessons they have learned along the way.

9.1 Personal Accounts of Breast Cancer Survivors

Every breast cancer journey is unique, and survivors have different experiences to share. These personal accounts provide valuable insights into the emotional and physical challenges faced by individuals diagnosed with breast cancer.

One survivor, Sarah, recalls the initial shock of her diagnosis. She can well recall the anxiety and apprehension that came with the news.
 However, through her treatment and support from loved ones, Sarah found strength within herself. She emphasizes the importance of a positive mindset and

the power of self-care during the recovery process.

Another survivor, Lisa, shares her story of overcoming adversity. She faced multiple setbacks during her treatment, including complications and the need for additional surgeries. Despite these challenges, Lisa remained determined and focused on her recovery. Her story serves as a reminder that resilience and perseverance can lead to eventual triumph.

9.2 Triumphs and Lessons Learned

Breast cancer survivors not only overcome physical challenges but also gain profound insights that shape their lives moving forward. Their triumphs and lessons learned offer guidance and inspiration to others facing similar journeys.

One common theme among survivors is the newfound appreciation for life. Many express gratitude for the simple joys and moments that were previously taken for granted. The experience of battling breast cancer often leads survivors to reevaluate their priorities and find a renewed sense of purpose.

Survivors also emphasize the importance of support systems. Family, friends, and support groups play a crucial role in providing emotional and practical assistance throughout the journey. The bonds formed during this challenging time can be transformative, creating lifelong connections and a sense of belonging.

Additionally, survivors highlight the significance of advocacy and spreading awareness. Breast cancer survivors often become passionate advocates, working to educate others about the disease, promote early detection, and support research initiatives. Their stories of hope and resilience inspire others to take action and contribute to the fight against breast cancer.

The uplifting tales of breast cancer survivors serve as beacons of hope and tenacity, to sum up. These personal accounts provide invaluable insights into the challenges faced by individuals diagnosed with breast cancer and the triumphs they achieve along the way. Through their experiences, survivors emphasize the importance of a positive mindset, self-care, support systems, gratitude, and advocacy. Their stories inspire others to remain hopeful, spread awareness, and support the fight against breast cancer.

Remember, you are not alone in this journey. Stay strong, stay positive, and join the community of survivors and advocates who are making a difference in the lives of those affected by breast cancer.

10 | Conclusion

Breast cancer is one of the most prevalent forms of cancer worldwide, affecting millions of individuals each year. As medical advancements continue to improve, it is crucial to emphasize the importance of continued breast cancer awareness. This conclusion section will explore the significance of raising awareness, highlighting the importance of early detection and providing support for those affected by breast cancer.

10.1 The significance of maintaining breast cancer awareness

Breast cancer awareness campaigns have played a pivotal role in educating communities about the risk factors, symptoms, and preventive measures associated with breast cancer. These initiatives aim to increase public understanding and knowledge, empowering individuals to take proactive steps towards their breast health. By promoting awareness, we can encourage regular self-examinations, clinical screenings, and early detection, leading to higher survival rates and improved treatment outcomes.

Raising awareness also helps dispel myths and misconceptions surrounding breast cancer. Many individuals still hold outdated beliefs about the disease, leading to delayed diagnosis and treatment. By providing accurate information, we can combat these misconceptions and promote a better understanding of breast cancer, ultimately saving lives.

Furthermore, continued breast cancer awareness is crucial in addressing disparities in healthcare access and outcomes. Certain communities, such as low-income populations and minority groups, face barriers to healthcare services, resulting in delayed diagnosis and inadequate treatment. By focusing on awareness campaigns, we can bridge these gaps, ensuring that everyone has equal access to early detection and quality care.

10.2 Encouragement for Early Detection and Support

Early detection is the key to successful breast cancer treatment. Encouraging individuals to be proactive in their breast health is essential for early diagnosis and improved prognosis. By promoting regular self-examinations and clinical screenings, we can empower individuals to detect any abnormalities promptly.

Breast self-examinations are simple, yet effective tools for early detection. Encouraging women and men to perform regular self-examinations can help them identify any changes in their breasts, such as lumps, skin changes, or nipple discharge. These self-examinations should be complemented by routine clinical screenings, including mammograms and ultrasounds, which can detect breast cancer even before symptoms arise.

Support is also a crucial aspect of breast cancer awareness. A breast cancer diagnosis can be emotionally and physically challenging, affecting not only the patient but also their loved ones. By fostering a supportive environment, we can provide comfort, encouragement, and resources to those affected by breast cancer. Support groups, counseling services, and educational programs can help individuals navigate the complexities of their diagnosis and treatment journey.

Conclusion

Continued breast cancer awareness is of paramount importance in our ongoing fight against this devastating disease. By raising awareness, we can empower individuals to take charge of their breast health, promoting early detection and improving treatment outcomes. It is crucial to address disparities in healthcare access and outcomes, ensuring that everyone, regardless of their socioeconomic background, has equal access to quality care.

Encouragement for early detection through self-examinations and clinical screenings is vital in detecting breast cancer at its earliest stages, leading to more successful treatment outcomes. Additionally, providing support to those affected by breast cancer is essential in helping them navigate the emotional and physical challenges that accompany a diagnosis.

In conclusion, by prioritizing continued breast cancer awareness, we can make significant strides in reducing the burden of this disease. Through education, early detection, and support, we can empower individuals, save lives, and work towards

a future where breast cancer is no longer
a life-threatening condition.

Afterword

Thank you for choosing to read "Breast Cancer Awareness." I sincerely hope that this book has provided you with valuable knowledge about breast cancer. If you have a moment, I would greatly appreciate it if you could take the time to leave a review at the store where you purchased it. Your feedback is incredibly important, as it can guide and support other readers who are searching for a trustworthy and informative resource on this life-threatening disease.

As an author, my ultimate goal is to create a comprehensive and empowering resource that enables individuals like yourself to embark on a transformative journey of awareness. Your insights and opinions can truly make a difference and provide invaluable guidance to others.

Once again, thank you for being a dear reader, and I hope our paths cross again within the pages of another captivating book.

Thank you for graciously considering our request. We are eagerly anticipating your valuable feedback, as your support holds immeasurable significance to us.